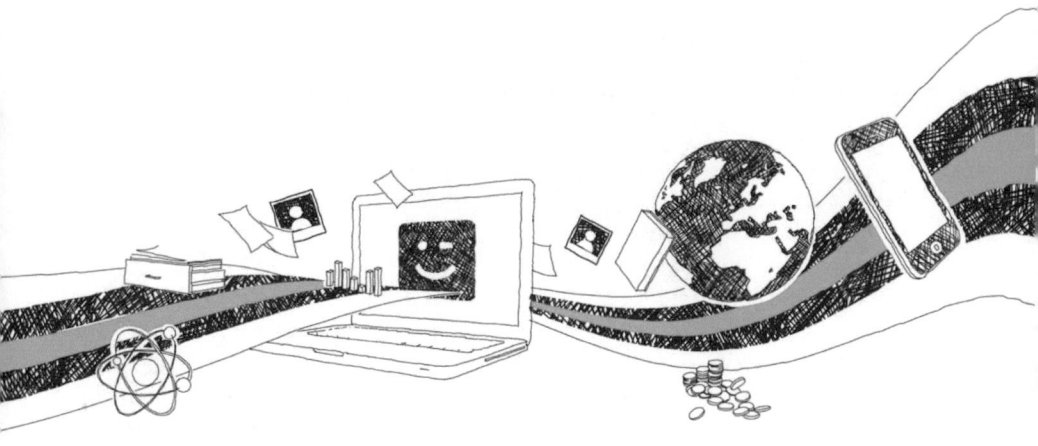

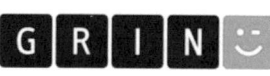

Imprint:

Copyright © 2013 GRIN Verlag, Open Publishing GmbH
Print and binding: Books on Demand GmbH, Norderstedt Germany
ISBN: 9783668400979

This book at GRIN:

http://www.grin.com/en/e-book/353857/a-critical-analysis-of-a-current-health-care-
policy-and-its-impact-on-a

Andrew Homer

A critical analysis of a current health care policy and its impact on a group of clients

GRIN Publishing

GRIN - Your knowledge has value

Since its foundation in 1998, GRIN has specialized in publishing academic texts by students, college teachers and other academics as e-book and printed book. The website www.grin.com is an ideal platform for presenting term papers, final papers, scientific essays, dissertations and specialist books.

Visit us on the internet:

http://www.grin.com/

http://www.facebook.com/grincom

http://www.twitter.com/grin_com

A critical analysis of a current health care policy and its impact on a group of clients/users

Submission Date   12/02/2013

Word Count   2700

The aim of this essay is to critically analyse the impact of smoke-free legislation and smoking cessation, as part of a wider anti-smoking strategy, on individuals admitted in an inpatient psychiatric setting. This will involve discussing the economic, ethical, legal and social influences that helped shape this policy as well as the physical and psychological impact on Patients. It will seek to explain how the views of patients and staff affect the implementation of this policy while discussing the effectiveness of interventions used under the policy. Some gaps in the legislation and policy will be discussed with recommendations as to how to address these and have a positive impact on the physical and mental health of patients in psychiatric settings.

The Department of Health (DH) (2012) estimates that illnesses caused by smoking cost the NHS £50,000,000 a week. The wider economic cost is said to be almost £14 billion a year. This is said to be made up of the cost of fires caused by smoking, loss of productivity from taking smoking breaks, employees who die from smoking related diseases and passive smoking. Some ethical issues, raised by charities such as Action on Smoking and Health (ASH), have had a significant role in the development of smoking policy and legislation. ASH (1997) argued that most smokers did not realise the full implications of smoking over a prolonged period of time and were unaware of the difficulties involved in trying to stop. They further argue that individuals who smoked were in actual fact not making an informed decision based on the full facts of smoking. This was said to be attributed to tobacco companies not doing enough to provide information on their products. Other ethical issues raised include the effects of passive smoking. Several studies have concluded that second hand smoke has a detrimental effect on the health of non-smokers and have raised the ethical issue of parents smoking around their children. (ASH, 1997)

The DH (1998) suggested a code of practice be created to help shield individuals in the workplace from passive smoking by creating non-smoking areas for individuals who didn't smoke. This would particularly apply to restaurants and bars. DH (2004) released another publication to enforce a ban on smoking in all public spaces and places of work however clubs and bars were exempt. This exemption was later removed and extended to all public spaces. ASH, 2011)

Changes in smoking policy were gradually introduced in light of evidence and reports by the World Health Organisation WHO (1999) and the Department of Health DH (2004) where it

2

was found that second hand smoke caused a detrimental effect on health. Recommendations from other organisations such as Action against Smoking Harm ASH and Cancer Research UK also contributed to smoke free policy. (ASH, 2011)

The Framework Convention on Tobacco Control (FCTC) is an international treaty which was created by the WHO as a response to the tobacco epidemic based on evidence of adverse health effects. It came into existence in 2005 to promote health and guidance from a legal aspect. The UK became an active member in 2004 and ever since has had obligations to carry out measures to address the tobacco epidemic. As a member of the FCTC the UK government is required to fulfil general obligations. These include creating local policies and safeguarding them from the tobacco industry, offering individuals help to stop smoking and protecting non-smokers from passive smoke.

With the introduction of the Health Act (2006) by the government the consensus among healthcare practitioners was that it would lower smoking rates and thus diseases caused by smoking (Jochelson, 2006). Smoke free legislation is part of a bigger anti-smoking strategy by the government which includes reducing the demand for tobacco through taxation and pricing, health warnings, advertising bans and smoking cessation.

Ratschen et al (2011) highlight the strong correlation between rates of smoking in mentally ill patients, estimating that about 50% of patients with depression or anxiety smoke. Furthermore it is estimated that 70% of patients diagnosed with schizophrenia are also smokers. It is believed that smoking is seen amongst some mental health practitioners as having a direct impact on physical health and therefore not fully their responsibility. Ratschen et al (2007) however argue that smoking can be categorised as a dependence syndrome, with chemicals in tobacco also interacting with antipsychotic medication. Nicotine in tobacco is also said to affect an individual's mood and thought process (Ratschen et al, 2007)

Jochelson (2006) argued that implementing smoking policy would be problematic but also saw it as allowing for a more comprehensive approach to administering care, allowing healthcare professionals to focus on both the mental and physical aspects of a client's health. Before legislation was enforced the three main issues debated were healthcare professionals exposure to second hand smoke, the patients' rights to freely choose their own lifestyle and their right to smoke and the impact this had on other patients. (Jochelson, 2006)

Stubbs et al (2004) conducted a study to examine the attitudes of mental health practitioners towards smoking in a psychiatric setting. They found that majority of the staff believed patients should have the right to smoke in assigned areas on the ward. They also believed that denying patients the right to smoke increased the likelihood of aggression. Campion et al (2008) also carried out a study whereby an outright smoking ban was implemented on a mental health unit. As a result of the smoking ban, staff members began escorting patients off the ward to smoke. Some staff were observed smoking with the patients. Staff members reported increasing levels of aggression towards themselves and due to this the study was discontinued after 2 weeks. Campion et al (2008) concluded that the outcome of the study was unknown due to its short lifespan and due to the fact that reports of aggression by patients and calls to end the study were made by staff who were themselves smokers. The results of this study suggested that effective implementation of smoking policy depends on staff compliance which could be a barrier. He also suggests that allowing concessions with regards to implementing smoking policy render it inconsistent and inefficient, thus making it fail. In order for it to succeed it would need to be implemented in a consistent way (Campion et al, 2008). Jochelson (2006) also argues that because most inpatient psychiatric units allow smoking in designated areas, the implications are that staff and patients are likely to be affected by passive smoking. Jochelson (2006) also concludes that policy makers have been selective by implementing smoking bans which does not make it effective. A possible cause of this selectiveness could be the fact that mental health units are not mentioned in the legislation. Influence and beliefs from patient advocates and some healthcare professionals also acts against the policy. There is the belief that smoking is the right of every individual even though Nice (2004) state that it is detrimental to patients both physically and financially. Others believe that every individual has the right to breathe in unpolluted air. These conflicting views make it difficult to implement the policy effectively and it ultimately has an impact on patients. (Jochelson, 2006)

One theme that can be taken from this study is Staff smoking with patients or even allowing patients to smoke in assigned areas could be seen as going against the NMC (2008) code of conduct which expects staff to promote good health and can be seen as negatively impacting on the patients' health.

Jochelson (2006) argues that most smokers would like to stop smoking but are unable to due to the existence of a culture within mental health settings and the belief that patients use tobacco as a form of self-medication to counter the effects of psychotic medication. (Kumari et al, 2005). Results from a study by Aguilar et al (2005) suggest that contrary to the belief that smoking has a therapeutic effect on symptoms of schizophrenia; there is actually a complex connection between nicotine dependence and the symptoms of schizophrenia. Aguilar et al (2005) concluded that more research was needed. Punnoose et al (2006) also found no evidence supporting this belief. Jochelson (2006) believes that only an outright ban will be effective as it will eliminate staff and patients being subjected to second hand smoke, not to mention the positive physical health benefits of smoking cessation.

One aspect of the partial ban in psychiatric settings is the ability for staff and patients to form therapeutic relationships with patients especially when supervising smoking in designated areas. However Lawn (2004) argues that the smoking culture in mental health units influences non-smoking patients and could possibly turn them into smokers. This culture shared by both patients and staff alike makes it difficult to reap the possible benefits of smoke free policy.

Individuals with mental Health problems are said to consume 42% of all cigarettes and tobacco and account for most deaths among this group in England. It is believed that most would like to stop but can only do so with good support DH (2011). It is reported that people with mental illnesses generally have a lower life expectancy than that of the general population. This coupled with smoking drastically lowers their life expectancy. Therefore one of the most important benefits of smoking cessation is an increased lifespan. This would suggest that Campion et al (2008) and Jochelson's (2006) recommendation for an outright ban is justified. If outright bans were introduced across the NHS it would complement the NMC (2008) code which asks for healthcare professionals to promote good health among patients. The current policy which still allows patients to smoke which means they are at a higher risk of diseases such as Lung cancer, chronic obstructive pulmonary disease and Pneumonia. In a study by Mcfall et al (2010) the introduction of smoking cessation treatment to patients who suffered from Post-Traumatic Stress Disorder led to larger numbers of patients quitting. However Mcfall et al (2010) argue that most mental health patients do not have receive smoking cessation interventions.

NICE (2004) stressed that independent smoking cessation services should be in constant communication with mental health workers and should be sharing information on patients who would like to stop smoking. They also stressed the need for nurses and other health care workers to continuously ask patients about their smoking habits and provide them with information on how to quit. Those that wished to stop smoking should then be referred to a smoking cessation specialist while remembering to monitor interactions with antipsychotic medications. This is due to reported cases where the levels of some antipsychotic medications in blood are influenced by smoking. More specifically, a patient prescribed Clozapine for instance, will have lower concentrations of the drug in their blood. Patients actively reducing the number of cigarettes they smoke will have an incremental effect on psychotropic medication plasma levels and therefore increased side effects. The dosage of medication would have to be lowered in this case. Derenne et al (2005) reported significantly higher levels of prescribed Clozapine in the blood of patients who suddenly stopped smoking. Ashir et al (2008) highlight the need to determine whether a patient smokes, before admission and to check the Clozapine blood concentration of patients on admission and upon discharge. (Ashir et al, 2008). NICE (2004) believed that compliance with these recommendations would help eradicate the smoking culture from psychiatric wards and create an environment that made it easier to stop smoking

Hughes (2007) found in a study that there was a strong relationship between suicide and smoking. He believed that smoking cessation can induce depression which can lead to suicidal thoughts and suicide. In contrast to this, a study by Malone (2003) of depressed smokers and non-smokers on a ward, found that the patients who smoked were more likely to carry out a suicide attempt. If this is the case then it would imply that this is an aspect of smoking policy that has not been addressed and in light of evidence, changes should be made (Malone, 2007). An implementation of Jochelson's (2006) suggestion to enforce an outright ban could address this.

Pharmacological methods of smoking cessation such as administration of Bupropion and Varenicline are said to be an effective way of reducing smoking rates in psychiatric patients, however it has also been found that these drugs can cause depression and lead to suicidal ideations as well. The Medicines and Healthcare products Regulatory Agency MHRA (2011) issued a warning advising against prescription of Bupropion to psychiatric patients due to reports of increased depression and aggression. Varenicline has also been reported to increase some symptoms of schizophrenia. MHRA (2011) advised of the need to closely monitor psychiatric patients who were prescribed Bupropion and for healthcare professionals to monitor any changes in mood. Consequently both Bupropion and Varenicline have several other possible unwanted side effects. (MHRA, 2011)

A review of studies found that counselling by nurses as part of smoking cessation treatments had a small but positive effect on reducing smoking rates among mental health patients. (Campion et al, 2008) Motivational interviewing when complemented with other pharmacological treatments was also found to be effective (Lai et al, 2010)

Smoke free policy has been shown to reduce the incidences of patients who are exposed to second hand smoke. There is also evidence of a slight reduction in smoking rates as a direct effect of smoke free policy. Significant improvements in physical health since the legislation have also been observed with increases in referrals of smokers and adherence to policy. (Callinan et al, 2010) This is in contrast to Campion et al's (2008) findings which reported compliance to be an important barrier to implementation of smoke free policy and legislation. It remains important for mental health professionals to be aware of patients who are smokers and if need be, to refer them to specialist smoking cessation services while keeping in mind the possible interactions with psychotropic medications. (NICE, 2004) In light of research, mental Health Workers should be aware of the possible suicidal effects of cigarettes on psychiatric patients and should monitor for changes in mood and possible aggression. (Hughes, 2007) Although Campion et al, (2008) reported an increase in patient aggression as a result of an outright ban on a psychiatric unit, Jochelson (2006) concluded that this was the most effective way of implementing smoke free policy as it would eliminate second hand smoke and allow staff to concentrate more on smoking cessation interventions.

References

Aguilar M, Gurpegui M, Diaz F, De Leon J (2005) Nicotine Dependence and Symptoms in Schizophrenia. British Journal of Psychiatry, 186:215-221

ASH (1997) Banning Tobacco Promotion: Ethical and Civil Liberties Issues. Accessed online at http://www.ash.org.uk/files/documents/ASH_168.pdf on 09/02/13

ASH (2011) Smoking and Respiratory Disease. Accessed online at http://ash.org.uk/files/documents/ASH_110.pdf on 09/02/13

Ashir M, Patterson L (2008) Smoking Bans and Clozapine Levels. Advances in Psychiatric Treatment 14:398-399

Callinan JE, Clarke A, Doherty K, Kelleher C (2010) Legislative Smoking Bans for Reducing Second-Hand Smoke: Exposure, Smoking Prevalence and Tobacco Consumption. The Cochrane Database of Systematic Reviews

Campion J, Lawn S, Brownlie A, Hunter E, Gynther B, Pols R (2008) Implementing Mental Smoke-Free Policies in Mental Health Inpatient Units: Learning from unsuccessful Experience. Australasian Psychiatry 16: 92

De Leon J, Diaz F (2005) A meta-analysis of worldwide studies demonstrates an association between schizophrenia and tobacco smoking behaviors. Schizophrenia Research, 76:135-157

Derenne J, Baldessarini R (2005) Clozapine Toxicity Associated With Smoking Cessation: Case Report 12(5):469-471

DH (1998) Smoking kills: a White Paper on tobacco. Department of Health, London

DH (2004) Choosing Health: Making Healthy Choices easier. Department of Health, London

DH (2011) No Health without Mental Health. Department of Health, London

DH (2011) The Impact of Smoke Free Legislation in England: Evidence Review. Department of Health, London

DH (2012) Reporting Instrument of the WHO Framework Convention on Tobacco Control. Accessed Online at http://www.who.int/fctc/reporting/party_reports/uk_2012_report.pdf on 09/02/2013

DH (2004) Second-hand smoke: Review of evidence since 1998. Scientific Committee on Tobacco and Health pp4

Hughes, J. R. (2007) Depression during tobacco abstinence. *Nicotine and Tobacco Research*, 9, 443–446

Jochelson J, Majrowski B (2006) Clearing the Air. Debating Smoke-Free Policies in Psychiatric Units. London: King's Fund

Jochelson, K. (2006) Smoke Free Legislation and Mental Health Units: The Challenges Ahead. British Journal of Psychiatry 189:479-480

Kumari V, Postma P.(2005) Nicotine Use in Schizophrenia: The Self Medication Hypotheses. Neuroscience and Biobehavioural Reviews 29(6):1021-1034.

Lai DTC, Cahill K, Qin Y, Tang JL (2010) Motivational interviewing for smoking cessation. *Cochrane Database of Systematic Reviews*

Lawn S (2004). Systemic barriers to quitting smoking among institutionalised public mental health service populations: a comparison of two Australian sites. International Journal of Social Psychiatry, 50:204-15

Malone K, Waternaux C, Haas G, Cooper T, Li S, Mann J (2003) Cigarette Smoking, Suicidal Behaviour and Serotonin Function in Major Psychiatric Disorders. American Journal of Psychiatry, 160:773-779

McFall M, Saxon A, Malte C, Chow B, Bailey S, Baker D, Beckham J, Boardman K, Carmody T, Joseph A, Smith M, Shih M, Lu Y, Holodniy M, Lavori P (2010) Integrating Tobacco Cessation into Mental Health Care for Posttraumatic Stress Disorder: A Randomized Controlled Trial 304(22):2485-2493

McNally L, Oyefeso A, Annan J, Perryman K, Bloor R, Freeman S, Wain B, Andrews H, Grimmer M, Crisp A, Oyebode D Ghodse A, (2006) A Survey of Staff Attitudes to Smoking-

Related Policy and Intervention in Psychiatric and General Health Care Settings. Journal of Public Health, 28(3):192-196

MHRA (2011) Guidance. Accessed Online at http://www.mhra.gov.uk/Safetyinformation/Generalsafetyinformationandadvice/Product-specificinformationandadvice/Product-specificinformationandadvice%E2%80%93M%E2%80%93T/Stopsmokingtreatments/index.htm on 09/02/13

NICE (2004) Smoking and Patients With Mental Health Problems. National Institute for Clinical Excellence. Accessed online at http://www.nice.org.uk/niceMedia/documents/smoking_mentalhealth.pdf on 09/02/13

Punnoose S, Belgamwar M (2006). Nicotine for Schizophrenia. The Cochrane Database of Systematic Reviews.

Ratschen E, Britton J and McNeill A (2009) Tobacco Dependence, Treatment and Smoke-Free Policies: A Survey of Mental Health Professionals' Knowledge and Attitudes. General Hospital Psychiatry, 31(6):576-582

Ratschen E, Britton J and McNeill A, (2009) Implementation of smoke-free policies in mental health in-patient settings in England. British Journal of Psychology. 194: 547-551

Ratschen E, Britton J and McNeill A, (2011) The Smoking Culture in Psychiatry: *Time for Change*. The British journal of Psychiatry 198: 6 – 7

WHO (1999) International Consultation on Environmental Tobacco Smoke (ETS) and Child Health. Tobacco Free Initiative, Accessed online at http://www.who.int/tobacco/research/en/ets_report.pdf on 09/02/13

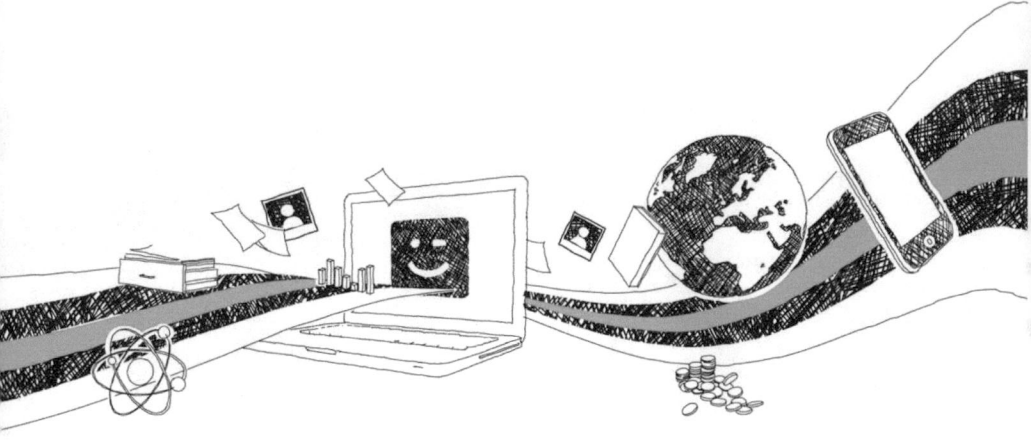
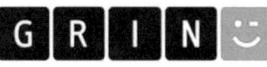